Headaches

Amazing All Natural Remedies to Alleviate Migraines, Cluster, Sinus, Tension and Rebound Headaches

Robert S. Lee

Contents

Chapter 1. A Look at Headaches & Their Causes

If you suffer from headaches and migraines on a regular basis, you may be wondering why. There are many causes for headaches and migraines, and there are also natural remedies that will help you to get rid of them. A headache is simply when your head hurts, and there can be many causes. You can get a headache from being hit in the head, but usually there is an internal reason why your head is hurting you.

A migraine is an acute headache, and it usually has to do with the swelling of the blood vessels, but there are many ways to get a migraine as well as to reduce it. You don't need to turn to over the counter medication or prescription drugs to get rid of headaches. Even chronic ones can be taken care of with natural remedies.

Some Basic Causes:

Dehydration is one of the leading causes of headaches, and it's a simple fix that many people don't think about. Drinking water can keep headaches at bay, but alcohol, soda, sweet tea, or other drinks that aren't hydrating can lead to dehydration without you even knowing.

You'll also find that inflammation can cause headaches, and there are many herbal remedies that can help. High blood pressure can also cause headaches and migraines, where your blood vessels are constricted, causing acute pain. Inflammation fighting foods and supplements can provide instant relief.

Stress can cause headaches as well, and there are many remedies in this book that will teach you how to get rid of your stress quickly and effectively. Anxiety will also cause headaches and migraines, but keeping anxiety and stress down on a regular basis can be tough when you're trying to do it without any help. Tension is also a leading cause of headaches and migraines, which can be worsened by stress and anxiety. Tension headaches can be difficult to get rid of, but tension can be reduced naturally as well.

Get Rid of Headaches Quickly:

The effectiveness of a natural or herbal remedy is dependent on how soon you recognize your headache symptoms so that you can treat them immediately. Try to keep headaches from turning into migraines, and then it'll be easier for you to get rid of. Natural remedies aren't nearly as effective if you don't know when to apply them. Preemptive measurements may also be taken to make sure that you do not develop a headache after a stressful day or even in a noisy situation.

Chapter 2. Headache & Migraine Relief Salves

There are many different salves that you can use for migraines and even normal headaches. It's easy to make sure that your headache goes away quickly. Salves are able to be carried around with you, and it helps to provide relief wherever you go. Of course, make sure that you have an airtight container, usually glass is best, so that you can store your salve effectively.

Salve #1 Solid Headache Salve

The main ingredient for this solid salve is lavender, but the peppermint essential oil is known to help with headaches as well. The coconut oil is great for your skin, and it acts a carrier oil, and keeps the recipe at a salve consistency. You can relieve tension with peppermint and lavender essential oil, helping with tension headaches quickly and effectively. The combination is soothing and easy to make.

Ingredients:

1. 1 Tablespoon Beeswax, Grated
2. 6 Tablespoons Coconut Oil
3. 4-6 Drops Lavender Essential Oil
4. 5-8 Drops Peppermint Essential Oil

Directions:

1. Melt your beeswax and coconut oil together in a double boiler on low. Stir gently to combine when melted, and stir in your essential oils.
2. Pour into containers and let cool before sealing.

Salve #2 Soft Migraine Salve

This is a salve that is a little softer, and so it applies a little easier. You'll notice that it also has lavender and peppermint essential oils to help target the tension that may be causing your headache, but basil essential is also known to help. Basil essential oil is known as a pain relief essential oil, and it takes effect rather quickly. Add more beeswax if you want a thicker salve to apply.

Ingredients

1. 7 Drops Lavender Essential Oil
2. 5 Drops Peppermint Essential Oil
3. 5 Tablespoons Coconut Oil
4. 4 Drops Basil Essential Oil
5. ½ Teaspoon Beeswax, Grated

Directions:

1. Take your beeswax and coconut oil putting it over low heat in a double boiler.
2. Once melted and mixed together, turn off the heat and mix in your essential oils. Make sure it is thoroughly mixed.
3. Pour into containers, and let firm up and cool down before sealing.

Salve #3 Chamomile & Lavender

Roman chamomile is yet another great essential oil to add to the mix for any headache and migraine, and this salve is soft and easy to apply. It has a floral scent with a fresh peppermint tinge, and the roman chamomile is known to calm down stress and anxiety as well, which can contribute to and worsen an already existing headache. It's also anti-inflammatory, and inflammation can contribute to a headache and keep it from going away.

Ingredients:

1. 10 Drops Roman Chamomile Essential Oil
2. 2-3 Drops Peppermint Essential Oil
3. 10-15 Drops Lavender Essential Oil
4. 1 Tablespoon Beeswax, Grated
5. 5 Tablespoons Coconut Oil

Directions:

1. Take your coconut oil and beeswax, melting in a double boiler over low heat to combine.
2. Turn heat off, and then add in all essential oils.
3. Pour into containers, and let firm and cool down before sealing.

Salve #4 Relaxing Headache Blend

The star in this wonderful headache blend is the eucalyptus. When paired with the lavender and peppermint for tension and then the basil for general pain and quick relief, you'll find that it works quickly. It has a slightly medicinal smell, but it still soothes mental fatigues and the headaches that come with them. If you're tired and need a little more clarity, then this would be the headache blend to use.

Ingredients:

1. 10 Drops Eucalyptus Essential Oil
2. 6 Drops Lavender Essential Oil
3. 5 Drops Peppermint Essential Oil
4. 8 Drops Basil Essential Oil
5. 1 Tablespoon Beeswax, grated
6. 4 Tablespoons Coconut Oil

Directions:

1. Melt your beeswax and coconut oil together over low heat in a double boiler before taking off heat and mixing in all essential oils.
2. Make sure it's well blended before pouring into containers to cool down and firm before sealing.

Salve #5 Magnesium Blended Soothing Salve

Magnesium is another great oil to use in a salve when you're looking for a way to quickly get rid of a nasty headache. If you have a healthy level of magnesium, you're much less likely to suffer from headaches in the first place, but the other essential oils provide immediate relief. The magnesium oil can help you in the long term, while the lemon essential oil helps to melt away any stress that could be causing tension and therefore the headache at hand. Of course, you can't forget castor oil since it provides natural pain relief.

Ingredients:

1. 1 Tablespoon Magnesium Oil
2. 20 Drops Peppermint Essential Oil
3. 10 Drops Lavender Essential Oil
4. 10 Drops Lemon Essential Oil
5. ½ Ounce Beeswax, Grated
6. 4 Tablespoons Extra Virgin Olive Oil
7. 2 Tablespoons Castor Oil

Directions:

1. Melt your beeswax in a double boiler, and then mix in your extra virgin olive oil. Take off heat to mix in all essential oils and magnesium oil.
2. Pour into containers and let cool before sealing.

Salve #6 Minty Relief

You already know that peppermint will help to soothe away even the worst headache and migraine, but in this combination it's going to work even better. Wintergreen essential oil also has a minty smell to it, and it's known as another general pain-reliever. Wild orange essential oil gives this blend a citrusy finish, and it relieves stress, anxiety, and helps you to relax so your headache will go away even faster.

Ingredients:

1. 15 Drops Wintergreen Essential Oil
2. 10 Drops Wild Orange Essential Oil
3. 10 Drops Peppermint Essential Oil
4. ¼ Cup Coconut Oil
5. 2 Tablespoons Beeswax, Grated

Directions:

1. Melt the beeswax and coconut oil together in a double boiler over low heat, and then add in essential oils.
2. Pour it into containers and let cool before sealing.

Salve #7 Numbing Relief Mix

This is a great blend, and it has many anti-inflammatory effects. You'll find that clove essential is a great numbing agent, even applied topically in this headache salve. The ginger essential oil adds more anti-inflammatory effects while wintergreen and peppermint work together to give long term relief while the headache completely dissipates. This is a very soft salve, and it goes on very similarly to lotion. For a more solid texture, more beeswax will be needed, and you'll want to add less coconut oil. A soft salve is usually best for this headache blend because it helps the clove to take effect quickly by soaking into your skin.

Ingredients:

1. 7 Drops Clove Essential Oil
2. 10 Drops Peppermint Essential Oil
3. 4 Drops Ginger Essential Oil
4. 10 Drops Wintergreen Essential Oil
5. 6 Teaspoons Coconut Oil
6. 1 Teaspoon Beeswax, Grated

Directions:

1. Heat your beeswax and coconut oil together. Remember to use a double boiler and put it over low heat.
2. When it's melted and thoroughly mixed, you can then add in essential oils and take off heat.
3. Pour into prepared containers and let cool and firm before sealing.

Salve #8 Clove & Lavender

Just remember that sometimes simple combinations can work the best, and that's exactly what this salve takes advantage of. With the relaxing scent of lavender to relieve stress and tension paired with the numbing agent and pain killer of the clove essential oil, this is an effective duo. A little goes along ways, but you may still want to use a little more if your headache has progressed or even if you're suffering from a migraine.

Ingredients:

1. 10 Drops Clove Essential Oil
2. 15-20 Drops Lavender Essential Oil
3. 4 Teaspoons Coconut Oil
4. 1 ½ Teaspoons Beeswax, Grated

Directions:

1. Take a double boiler and put it over low heat before adding in your beeswax and coconut oil. Let melt over low heat, stirring together.
2. Add in essential oils as you take off heat, and pour into containers to cool and firm before sealing.

Salve #9 Relaxing Headache Rub

Spearmint essential oil has been added to this minty blend, and the roman chamomile will help to relax you while the spearmint does its job. It's a quick external agent to help relieve inflammation and tension so that your headache can disappear in no time at all. This is a rub that is known to have a slightly medicinal scent to it.

Ingredients:

1. 10 Drops Spearmint Essential Oil

2. 5 Drops Peppermint Essential Oil

3. 10 Drops Eucalyptus Essential Oil

4. 7 Drops Roman Chamomile Essential Oil

5. ¼ Cup Coconut Oil

6. 2 Teaspoons Beeswax, Grated

Directions:

1. Melt your beeswax in a double boiler over low heat before adding in your coconut oil, making sure to stir to combine before adding in all essential oils.

2. Take off heat, and pour into containers. Remember to let them cool before sealing.

Salve #10 Nighttime Headache Relief

This is a salve that is best used at night, and it's because both the lavender and roman chamomile is meant to relax you and allow you to release tension. It's known to not only help you to get rid of a headache, but it can also be effective in helping you to get to sleep as well. Of course, you'll find that the helichyrsum essential oil also plays an important role because of its anti-inflammatory properties. This salve is neither extremely soft nor solid, and it'll spread easily whenever you need to apply it.

Ingredients:

1. 8 Drops Roman Chamomile Essential Oil
2. 10 Drops Lavender Essential Oil
3. 15 Drops Helichyrsum Essential Oil
4. 2 Teaspoons Beeswax, Grated
5. 4 Tablespoons Coconut Oil

Directions:

1. Take a double boiler and put it over low, adding in your beeswax and your coconut oil. Make sure that they mix together while melting, and then add in your essential oils. Stir to combine.
2. Pour into containers, and then let cool before you seal them up to use later.

Chapter 3. Essential Oil Blends that Really Help

If you know how to blend essential oils, then you will be able to get a blend that is going to help you to relax and get rid of your headache fast. These blends will help you to feel better quickly, and they're easy to make. Just make sure that you have a carrier oil to top the blend off with and put them in rollerball bottles so that you can carry them with you and use them whenever you need them.

Essential Oil Blend #1 Sinus Headache

Eucalyptus and peppermint is another minty and medicinal duo to help. The peppermint will help with inflammation but so will the eucalyptus. Both helps your body to relax, and it's even known as a decongestant, which is what makes it useful for treating sinus related headaches. You can apply it to your temples or around your nose. You should notice immediate relief, but stronger relief will come with time.

Ingredients:

1. 10 Drops Eucalyptus Essential Oil
2. 20 Drops Peppermint Essential Oil
3. Sweet Almond Oil

Directions:

1. Mix all essential oils together in the rollerball bottle and top off with sweet almond oil.

Essential Oil Blend #2 Fast Headache Relief

Frankincense is an essential oil that many people skip over, but that should never happen if you're looking for something to help with the pain in your head. It can help with your mood swings and fatigue as well. Frankincense can even help to lower your blood pressure, keep your stress under control, and relieve the pain of arthritis because of its anti-inflammatory effects. With the soothing effects of lavender, you'll find that this remedy works quickly but may make you sleepy. The peppermint is a stimulant, but you may still feel some sedative effects from the other two oils.

Ingredients:

1. Coconut Oil
2. 10 Drops Frankincense Essential Oil
3. 10 Drops Peppermint Essential Oil
4. 10 Drops Lavender Essential Oil

Directions:

1. Add all oil together in the rollerball bottle and mix. Shake before using so nothing settles or separates.

Essential Oil Blend #3 Bedtime Headaches

Vetiver oil is an essential oil that most people don't even know about, but it's still quite useful. It'll even help you to get to sleep while getting rid of your headache. It's best to use this salve before bed, and remember that it will help with mood swings, fatigue, stress, and inflammation. It'll even help to relieve your tension to make sure your headache is truly gone.

Ingredients:

1. 10 Drops Lavender Essential Oil
2. 10 Drops Vetiver Essential Oil

3. 10 Drops Frankincense Essential Oil
4. Sweet Almond Oil

Directions:

1. Mix all oils together in a rollerball bottle, shaking before each use so nothing separates.

Essential Oil Blend #4 Citrus Headache Blend

You already know that this is an essential oil blend that is meant to target the cause of your headache and eliminate it quickly. It's also a mood stabilizer and can help to melt the stress away from your day. It's good to use during any time of the day, and it's safe to carry with you despite the strong lavender scent, as it shouldn't make you sleepy.

Ingredients:

1. 5 Drops Frankincense Essential Oil
2. 10 Drops Lemon Essential Oil
3. 5 Drops Wild Orange Essential Oil
4. 15 Drops Lavender Essential Oil
5. Coconut Oil

Directions:

1. Mix everything together in the rollerball bottle, and make sure to shake before you use it.

Essential Oil Blend #5 Migraine & Headache Blaster

Wintergreen is your natural pain killer in this headache blaster, but birch essential oil still plays an essential role while the peppermint and lavender make sure that nothing is adding on to your already painful headache or migraine. Birch is also a natural pain reliever, and it's known to be quite powerful. When you combine it with the wintergreen, it'll help to make sure that you don't suffer for longer than necessary.

Ingredients:

1. 30 Drops Peppermint Essential Oil
2. 10 Drops Birch Essential Oil
3. 10 Drops Wintergreen Essential Oil
4. 30 Drops Lavender Essential Oil
5. Coconut Oil

Directions:

1. Mix all oils together before putting in a glass roller bottle, remember to top off with the coconut oil.

Essential Oil Blend #6 Headache Busting Blend

Geranium makes an appearance in this blend, but you'll find that almost all of the essential oils are equal. They all target different causes of your headaches while lavender is half because it will simply help with the stress that is making it work while having am mild sedative effect. It's also known to help with stress while relieving your tension pain nearly immediately.

Ingredients:

1. 8 Drops Helichrysum Essential Oil
2. 8 Drops Geranium Essential Oil

3. 8 Drops Frankincense Essential Oil
4. 4 Drops Lavender Essential Oil
5. 8 Drops Peppermint Essential Oil
6. Coconut Oil

Directions:

1. Blend all essential oils together and then top with coconut oil to fill up the rest of the rollerball bottle. Shake well before using.

Essential Oil Blend #7 Diffuser Headache Relief

You'll find that this earthy blend has a lot of new essential oils to bring to the table, such as marjoram which is sure to help. Marjoram essential oil is used for both toothaches and headaches as it's a powerful pain reliever. Thyme is also a great addition because it relieves stress, dizziness, and can even promote a healthy sleep cycle. When you aren't getting enough sleep or at least enough quality sleep, then you are much more likely to develop a migraine or headache during the day. Rosemary is another earthy essential oil that has been added so that your headache is relieved quickly. It has a soothing effect on the mind and body, while it still helps with headaches by making sure to treat tension.

Ingredients:

1. 15 Drops Marjoram Essential Oil
2. 15 Drops Thyme Essential Oil
3. 15 Drop Peppermint Essential Oil
4. 15 Drops Lavender Essential Oil
5. 15 Drops Rosemary Essential Oil

Directions:

1. Blend them together in an empty bottle, and then put ten drops into the diffuser

and keep the rest for later. Relax near your diffuser.

Essential Oil Blend #8 Earthy Headache Blend

Relieve your stress, help with inflammation, erase tension, and numb your headache pain quickly with this earthy essential oil blend. The only need addition is the bergamot, which will work wonders to help you. Most headaches or migraines are actually triggered by stress, which is what bergamot is great at helping you to deal with quickly.

Ingredients:

1. 15 Drops Thyme Essential Oil
2. 15 Drops Rosemary Essential Oil
3. Coconut Oil
4. 15 Drops Bergamot Essential Oil
5. 4 Drops Eucalyptus Essential Oil

Directions:

1. Mix all essential oils together, putting them in a glass rollerball bottle, and then top with coconut oil.
2. Shake well before each use.

Essential Oil Blend #9 Sandalwood Headache Blend

Let the clove essential oil numb your headache while your mood is lifted and your tension slips away. Sandalwood oil is the new edition to this essential oil blend, helping with inflammation and helping to keep your emotions in check. Without stress adding on to it continuously, it's much easier to get rid of your headache or migraine and actually keep it gone.

Ingredients:

1. 15-20 Drops Sandalwood Essential Oil

2. 10 Drops Thyme Essential Oil
3. 5 Drops Clove Essential Oil
4. 5 Drops Rosemary Essential Oil
5. Coconut Oil

Directions:

1. Mix all essential oils together before putting it in the rollerball bottle, and then top off with coconut oil. Shake before use.

Essential Oil Blend #10 Relaxation Blend

This is yet another simple blend that can actually work wonders, and every essential oil used in this blend is considered to be both affordable and relaxing. The roman chamomile will help to promote a healthy sleep cycle and erase stress immediate, while lavender melts your tension away. If you're worried that your headache may be caused by any inflammation, that's what the ginger essential oil is there for. They're all easy to find, and this blend is meant to be easy to make.

Ingredients:

1. 15 Drops Roman Chamomile Essential Oil
2. 10 Drops Lavender Essential Oil
3. 6 Drops Ginger Essential Oil
4. Coconut Oil

Directions:

1. Add all essential oils into the rollerball bottle, and then top with coconut and shake well.

Chapter 4. Bath Time Recipes to Work Quickly

Bath time is a relaxing time, and hot baths are actually known to help you with relaxation and stress relief, which can help to keep away headaches naturally. Of course, you can increase that relief and make sure to run a bath that really will get rid of your headache or migraine quickly with these bath time recipes. You'll find that they're easy to make, and even easier to use.

Bath Time Recipe #1 Peppermint Salts

A relaxing bath will usually make the difference, but you'll find that sometimes you only need a single essential oil added to some salts to make the difference in your bath. Epsom salts are specifically added in to help you to release the tension that you're feeling. Built up tension in your muscles will cause aggravation, stress, and even headaches. The peppermint is meant to soothe you and put your emotions back in order. You can use it for a headache, but it'll also help to improve your mood after a long day.

Ingredients:

1. 1 ½ Cups Epsom Salts
2. ½ Cup Sea Salt, Coarse
3. 30-40 Drops Peppermint Essential Oil

Directions:

1. Mix all of your salts together, and then add in the peppermint essential oil. Make sure it's thoroughly mixed before

putting in a glass jar. You can add more peppermint essential oil if you're looking for a stronger scent.

2. Take a handful and put it in your baht every time you need to get rid of a headache.

Bath Time Recipe #2 Lavender & Mint Scrub

It's easy to get ahold of lavender and peppermint. They're also a floral and minty scrub that will help you to exfoliate your skin while cleaning away your headache as well as your stress. It's a bath time recipe that is usually best to use in the evenings, as it can cause you to get sleepy and it'll promote a higher quality of sleep as well. The body can release natural tension while you're sleeping, which will assure that you don't wake up with another headache as well.

Ingredients:

1. ¼ Cup Sweet Almond Oil
2. 2 Cups Epsom Salts
3. 20 Drops Lavender Essential Oil
4. ½ Cup Lavender Buds, Dried
5. 15-20 Drops Peppermint Essential Oil

Directions:

1. Put your dried lavender buds into a blender and blend into a powder.
2. Add all ingredients together and mix before placing into an airtight glass jar for storage. Add a handful to your bath every time you need to get a headache.

Bath Time Recipe #3 Eucalyptus Salt Scrub

Eucalyptus and peppermint are a great scrub to go together, but usually you can't get ahold of the plants themselves. Of course, this is where the essential oil is a little easier to use. You can use Epsom salts for an added bonus if you want to make sure that you muscles aren't sore when you go to bed, and it'll help to make sure tension and stress doesn't contribute to the headache you already have or cause one later. Of course, the sea salt is a great exfoliator. You can use fine sea salt if you have delicate skin.

Ingredients:

1. 1 Cup Sea Salt, Coarse
2. 20 Drops Eucalyptus Essential Oil
3. 10 Drops Peppermint Essential Oil
4. ¼ Cup Coconut Oil

Directions:

1. Mix everything together, making sure that your coconut oil is melted first.

Bath Time Recipe #4 Earthy Sugar Scrub

This is a bath time recipe that is a bit more tedious to make. The Epsom salts will release tension, and the sugary scent is known to lighten your mood, just like with the rosemary and thyme. The lavender will relieve anxiety and stress, and you can use it in a bath soak as well. If you're using it in a bath soak, just remember to substitute the white sugar for sea salt.

Ingredients:

1. 15 Drops Rosemary Essential Oil
2. 15 Drops Thyme Essential Oil
3. 2 Tablespoons Thyme, Dried
4. ½ Cup Lavender Buds, Dried
5. ½ Cup Coconut Oil
6. 1 Cup Epsom Salts
7. ½ Cup White Sugar, Medium to Coarse

Directions:

1. Take your coconut oil and put it in a small saucepan, melting it and then add all of your essential oils.
2. Grind up the thyme, mixing it into the white sugar, and then add in the coconut oil mixture after you take it off heat. Add in Epsom salts, and then place it in a glass container that's airtight.

Bath Time Recipe #5 Chamomile & Rose Bath Salts

Rose isn't something that most people think of when they're looking for something to relieve them of pain, even head pain. However, it should be on the top of your list. It's meant to relax you and relieve both anxiety and stress, which in turn will light your headache drastically while the chamomile helps to relax you as well. They're a potent duo when put together, and using the rose petals makes this bath salt recipe a little more interesting and presentable. You can even use it as a gift.

Ingredients:

1. ½ Cup Rose Petals, Dried
2. 5 Drops Rose Essential Oil
3. 10 Drops Chamomile Essential Oil
4. ¼ Cup Chamomile Flowers, Dried
5. 1 Cup Epsom Salts

Directions:

1. Take a mortar and pestle, grinding your chamomile flowers and roses together, and mix in the Epsom salts.
2. Add in all essential oils, making sure to mix well. Use a handful whenever you need headache relief.

A Few Bath Time Tips:

You'll find that even though a nice bath with many of the recipes above will help you to get rid of a headache, it doesn't quite always work. There are many things you might be doing wrong when trying to clear your headache away when using a bath time solution. When you do everything right, you should be able to experience more relief from the remedies above, helping to ease away your migraine or headache.

Avoid bringing anything into the bathroom with you that requires concentration or your attention. You should be clearing your head and keeping yourself from focusing if you want the best results from the recipes above. This includes your phone, music, or even a book. These aren't needed when you're trying to relax, and they can strain your eyes, stress you out, and ruin the remedy that you've worked so hard to create.

Keeping the temperature warm is also important when you're looking for a bath time remedy for headaches and even migraines. Many headaches and migraines are caused by or furthered by stress, and you'll find that your body won't relax and release built up tension if the water is to cool. Many people will experience similar problems if the water is too hot. Make sure that the water is just right for you, and many people prefer it a little hotter in the beginning so that it can cool to the right temperature, helping it to stay at that temperature for the majority of your bath.

Remember that giving time for the remedy to work is also important. Some people will notice immediate results, but this is not the majority of people. The majority of people must soak for twenty to forty minutes before seeing results, and results will vary. It depends on how bad your migraine or headache is before you get into the bath on how much it will improve.

Chapter 5. Supplements as a Preemptive Strike

Supplements can be extremely important as a preemptive way to help keep chronic headaches and migraines at bay, but of course remember to talk to your doctor before adding any supplement to your daily routine. Supplements, even natural ones, can interact with medication whether it's over the counter or prescription. Make sure that your doctor knows of any prescription medication that you're taking as well.

Some supplements you are able to take on a daily basis as a preemptive way to help keep away headaches, but often others will help to get rid of your headache immediately. Some supplements are only able to be taken for a short period of time, but your doctor can advise you on what dosage to take, as even a supplement's recommended dosage may not be best for everyone.

Supplement #1 Butterbur

Butterbur is a supplement that is known for helping with headaches and migraines. It's considered to be anti-inflammatory herb, and it's effective to treat a headache as it's beginning to start. It's usually recommended that you take seventy-five milligrams of butterbur twice daily for the best effects, but it will not help much if your headache has already turned into a migraine that has set in. However, it can still help to lessen the pain as you use other natural salves or bath time recipes to help finish getting rid of it.

Supplement #2 Magnesium

You'll find that magnesium is also a natural supplement that you can take daily, and it will help to reduce the frequency that you have headaches or migraines. It helps to calm your nerves, and nerves can be commove overexcited when a headache or migraine starts. If you have chronic headaches or migraines, you may already be low in magnesium. Your doctor can test you for a magnesium deficiency, and they can help you to make sure that you have the right amount of magnesium to help you prevent your migraines.

Supplement #3 Vitamin D

Vitamin D is an easy vitamin to get ahold, and it can make the world of difference. Sadly, many people are becoming vitamin D deficiency, and it can come from spending too much time avoiding the sun or jus indoors. It can actually make you perceive pain to a higher degree if you're low in vitamin D. many doctors will recommend two thousand milligrams daily for the best results, but you can find out if you're vitamin D deficient by asking your doctor to run a simple blood test.

Supplement #4 Vitamin B2

Taking a vitamin B complex is usually best, but vitamin B2 can help you to make sure that you aren't going to have headaches or migraines as frequently. Vitamin B12, found in a vitamin B complex, will help to boost your energy levels as well, and it'll help you to feel better sooner. B2 reduces the frequency of migraines or general headaches.

Supplement #5 Feverfew

Feverfew is another herbal supplement that is known to help you with headaches. It will also help with nausea and even motion sickness. Of course, it's known to help with fevers. Feverfew is safe to take daily, and it can reduce the frequency of headaches you get. However, remember that you cannot take feverfew if you are allergic to ragweed, chamomile, or yarrow.

You should also not take feverfew if you're diabetic or have liver disease.

Supplement #6 Coenzyme Q10

You'll find that taking 150 milligrams of Coenzyme Q10 will help you to cut the amount of migraines and headaches you have on a regular basis in up to half. Of course, many people believe that you get better results by taking one hundred milligrams three times daily. To determine how much you should take or if coenzyme Q10 is for you, you need to talk to your doctor.

Supplement #7 Ginger

Some people have found that your frequency of headaches can be decreased by taking ginger on a regular basis. Many people do not get enough ginger in their daily diet to get the same effect by just adding it to their food, which is where a supplement comes in handy. It can also help with inflammation and nausea. It can stop inflammation and your migraine or headache in its track. For many people, it's fine to follow the directions on the bottle when taking ginger supplements.

Some Extra Help:

If you're looking for a way to take some of the above supplements with a little more pizzazz than just a supplement, then try a natural homemade gummy. These two gummy recipes are fun to take, and they can be taken on a regular basis to help make sure that you're controlling your headaches and keeping them at bay in a fun way.

Magnesium Gummies:

Magnesium is beneficial to your overall healthy, and it can be easy to make a tasty magnesium gummy that you take right before bed. It can even help to promote better sleep, which will help to keep migraines and headaches away.

Ingredients:

1. ¾ Cup Apple Juice
2. 3 Tablespoons Gelatin
3. 5 Tablespoons Magnesium Powder
4. 1 Tablespoon Honey, Raw

Directions:

1. Take the magnesium powder, and whisk it together with the cold juice until it is completely dissolved. You will need to give it a moment so that all of the bubbles go down, and then you can mix in the gelatin.
2. Heat up the mixture and continue to stir until it dissolves. It will clump at first, but you'll need to keep stirring.
3. Add in your honey, and mix well before taking it off heat.

4. Pour into silicon gummy molds, and put it in the fridge for an hour. Pop them out, and then keep them in the fridge in an airtight container. Many people use a Mason jar.

Ginger Gummies:

There are many different recipes for ginger gummies, but you'll find that they're easy to take, and they don't always have to taste of ginger too strongly. With honey, you'll find that this lemon and ginger gummy is sweet, and it can even help to boost your immune system and metabolic rate.

Ingredients:

1. 2 Teaspoons Grated Ginger, Fresh
2. 6 Tablespoons Honey, Raw
3. 2/3 Cup Lemon Juice, Fresh
4. 6 Tablespoons Gelatin Powder

Directions:

1. Take your lemon juice, ginger, and honey together in a saucepan, and whisk together. Sprinkle your gelatin over the top, and then whisk well before putting over medium heat.

2. Make sure to whisk constantly, and then let it come to a simmer. Let it simmer until you see it thicken and the gelatin completely dissolves. Once it's completely dissolved, you'll find that the mixture is clear and you can remove it from heat.

3. Pour into an eight by eight inch pan, or you can pour it into candy molds. Let cool completely in the fridge, and then you can cut them into pieces or pop them out of the molds. Store in the fridge and take one or two twice daily to help cut down with your headaches.

Chapter 6. Foods to Keep Headaches at Bay

You can use the right diet to help keep headaches at bay as well, and it'll help if you add these helpful foods into your diet on a regular basis if you want to make sure that you cut your headaches in half. It can be easy to add them into your diet, but you'll find an example of how to do so paired with each food. Remember that there are foods that can actually trigger headaches, and keeping a food log will help you to recognize those triggers so that you can start to cut them out of your diet. Skipping meals can also trigger migraines, so make sure that you stick to a schedule and eat at least three meals a day or six small meals daily.

Food #1 Watermelon

Watermelon is always a fun food to eat, and it's quite easy to put into your diet because you can eat it on its own. Watermelon helps with migraines and headaches because dehydration is a leading cause of headaches. When you're putting watermelon into your diet, you're helping your body to hydrate in a tasty way, and it'll help you to get rid of your headache a little quicker. Remember that many over the counter pills to help with headaches will actually dehydrate you more.

Example Recipe: Watermelon Chiller

This is a chilled watermelon drink that will help you to get watermelon into your system a little quicker. You can sweeten it with honey if need be, but many people find that you don't need to sweeten it at all.

Ingredients:

1. 2 Cups Watermelon, Seedless & Cubed
2. ½ Cup Coconut Water
3. 1 Teaspoons Honey, Raw

Directions:

1. Just pop everything in the blender together and blend until smooth. You can add ice if needed, but if your watermelon is cool you have a great juice.

Food #2 Coffee

A cup of coffee is actually known to help with a headache as well. However, remember that it only works in moderation. If you take too much coffee, then you'll become dehydrated which will also cause a headache. Coffee can actually help to relieve the size of your blood vessels and help your headache to go away.

Example Recipe: Simple Coffee

If you're looking to make the best coffee, then this recipe is going to help you. Remember that two much sugar can be counterproductive, so keep it to a minimum. Try a dairy free creamer as well, as it'll calm your stomach and help to make sure you have what you need to sweeten everything. Dairy can actually aggravate many headaches. Get your coffee maker ready and start brewing.

Ingredients:

1. 3 Tablespoons Coffee Grounds
2. 2 Teaspoons Non Dairy Creamer
3. 1 Teaspoons Cane Sugar

Directions:

61

1. Run your coffee through your coffee maker, and then add in your creamer and cane sugar, making sure it's mixed well before you drink it.

Food #3 Spinach

Spinach is going to help to relieve headaches and reduce their frequency as well. It's easy to add spinach into your diet, and it'll help to decrease your blood pressure so that your headache can go away on its own naturally or keep it away to begin with. You can replace most everything you use lettuce with spinach, helping you to get it into your diet and keep your blood pressure under control.

Example Recipe: Pear & Spinach Salad

This pear and spinach salad will help you to make sure that you're getting the spinach you need. Spinach salad is a great way to add in spinach in your daily routine, and it pairs with fruit very well. However, you can always eat spinach on its own as well.

Ingredients:

1. 1 Tablespoon Honey
2. ½ Teaspoon Sea Salt, Fine
3. 5 Cups Baby Spinach
4. 1 Medium Pear, Sliced Thin
5. 1 Tablespoon Olive Oil, Extra Virgin
6. ¼ Red Onion, Sliced Thin
7. 2 Tablespoons Red Wine Vinegar

Directions:

1. Take the onion, pear, and spinach and toss it in a bowl.
2. Combine the vinegar, salt, and honey together in a bowl. Mix in water if needed to thin, and then sprinkle over the salad as a natural dressing.

Food #4 Sesame Seeds

Sesame seeds are easy to use in various recipes, and they'll help to soothe a headache away as well. Many people will even add them to their smoothies to help sneak them into your diet in an easy way. The reason that sesame seeds help with your headache is because they are rich in vitamin E and can help to stabilize hormones. This can help women who suffer from headaches that are brought on by their menstrual cycles.

Example Recipe: Sesame Snaps

These are a hard sesame bar that taste sweet and will help you to get the sesame you need into your diet. Honey is the natural sweetener, and it can help with any sweet tooth or cravings that you might be having as well.

Ingredients:

1. ½ Cup Sesame Seeds
2. ½ Cup Sugar, White
3. 2 Tablespoons Honey, Raw

Directions:

1. Take two big sheets, placing wax paper over them and rub a little bit of vegetable oil on the wax paper as well. You'll want to dry roast the sesame seeds first, using a nonstick pan over low heat. You'll need to stir to make sure that you're the seeds

do not burn by stirring regularly. Make sure they're a golden color before transferring them to a place. You can use a little extra virgin olive oil if necessary to brown.

2. Take a pot, mixing in your honey and sugar, and then place it over medium heat and let it come to a boil. You'll need to mix constantly. Once it bubbles, cook for two minutes before you remove it from heat. Add in your sesame seeds, making sure it's blended well, and then put it on the wax paper.

3. Use a rolling pin to flatten out the mixture and let it harden.

4. Cut the bars apart, and they're ready to serve.

Food #5 Almonds

Almonds are great for headaches as well, and if you're experiencing one you may want to take a handful and eat them as a snack. The reason almonds can help to decrease your headache or migraine is because they are full of magnesium. Eating them on a regular basis will keep these headaches away for the same reason. It will help to relax your blood vessels as well.

Example Recipe: Cinnamon Roasted Almonds

Cinnamon roasted almonds are tasty, and they still have the magnesium you need to get rid of your headache quickly and effectively. Of course, it'll help to satisfy your taste buds as well. Add more cinnamon if desired.

Ingredients:

1. 1 Egg White
2. 1 Teaspoon Water, Cold

3. 3 Tablespoons Brown Sugar
4. 2 Teaspoons Honey, Raw
5. 1 Tablespoon Cinnamon, Ground
6. ¼ Teaspoon Sea Salt, Fine

Directions:

1. Preheat your oven to 250 degrees, and then beat your egg white in a bowl with the water until it's frothy. You'll then want to add in your almonds to stir and coat.
2. Mix in your honey, brown sugar, salt, and cinnamon together. Drizzle it over the nuts, making sure it's coated well.
3. Make sure to spread the almonds over a baking sheet that's been covered in parchment paper.
4. You'll want to roast the almonds for an hour, and make sure to stir every twenty minutes.

5. Allow to cool and then store or eat as desired.

Food #6 Bananas

Bananas are easy to eat on their own, and they'll help you to soothe a migraine or headache away. They'll even help to cure a hangover headache with no problems at all due to the potassium level. They're also high in magnesium to relax your blood vessels and help with all other headache and migraines.

Example Recipe: Cinnamon Banana Pops

This is a cool way to get the bananas you need, and you only need to make sure that you have Popsicle sticks and wax paper. Make sure that you have time to let them freeze, and then you can enjoy them at any time.

Ingredients:

1. 1 Tablespoon Honey, Raw
2. 1 Teaspoon Cinnamon, Ground
3. 1 Large Banana, Peeled

Directions:

1. Stick the Popsicle stick in the banana, and then coat with honey and sugar. Put on wax paper in the freezer, and let freeze before eating.

Chapter 7. Bonus Smoothie Recipes to Help

One great way to get what you need into your body to help relieve a headache naturally is by using a smoothie recipe to do it. You'll find that smoothie recipes are fun and easy, and headache crushing smoothie recipes are no different. So long as you know what type of ingredients to use, your headaches can be a thing of the past while you enjoy a wonderful drink.

Smoothie #1 Boosted Fruit Smoothie

You'll find that this smoothie recipe is boosted with rosemary to help you get over your headache fast. Of course, you already know that bananas will help as well. It stimulates the nerves and even helps to improve your circulation. It can help with cluster headaches, and it's easy to grow. Using fresh rosemary is usually best.

Ingredients:

1. 2 Large Bananas, Frozen & Sliced
2. ¼ Cup Strawberries
3. 1 Tablespoon Honey, Raw
4. ¼ Cup Rosemary, Fresh
5. ½ Cup Ice

Directions:

1. Blend everything together, and then drink while cool.

Smoothie #2 Banana & Coconut Twist

Yogurt is actually going to help you to get rid of a headache due to its high calcium content, and Greek yogurt is usually best. It helps to relax your body, and the banana and honey will help as well. It's even hydrating, which will help you to make sure that your headache isn't from dehydration.

Ingredients:

2. 1 Cup Coconut Milk, Chilled
3. ½ Cup Greek Yogurt, Vanilla
4. 1 Large Banana, Frozen & Sliced
5. ½ Cup Mango, Chunked & Frozen

Directions:

1. Just blend everything together, and then drink up.

Smoothie #3 Almond Butter Delight

Almonds give you the magnesium that you need to make sure that your headache goes away fast. Make sure that you have organic almond butter or at least one that doesn't have added sugar. This smoothie will give you that needed boost to chase your headache away.

Ingredients:

1. ½ Cup Almond Butter, Organic
2. 2 Teaspoons Honey, Raw
3. ½ Cup Coconut Water, Frozen
4. 1 Teaspoons Vanilla Extract
5. ½ Cup Spinach
6. 1 Medium Banana, Frozen & Sliced

Directions:

1. Just mix everything together in the
    blender, and blend until smooth.

Smoothie #4 Watermelon Delight

This hydrating mix is everything you need, and
you even add in sesame seeds to help make sure
that you have the right foods to keep your
migraine and headaches away.

Ingredients:

1. 2 Cups Watermelon, Cubed & Seedless
2. ½ Cup Greek Yogurt, Vanilla
3. 2 Tablespoons Sesame Seeds
4. 2 Tablespoons Honey, Raw
5. ¼ Cup Strawberries

Directions:

1. Blend everything on high in your blender until smooth, and then drink.

Smoothie #5 Ginger Blend

Ginger smoothies are a great way to help make sure that you have what you need to release inflammation and keep headaches and migraines away. Of course, just because you're using a ginger smoothie, it doesn't mean that it has to be bitter or even spicy.

Ingredients:

1. 1 ½ Cup Pineapple, Cubed & Chilled
2. 1 Small Banana, Frozen & Sliced
3. ½ Cup Greek Yogurt, Vanilla
4. 1 Tablespoon Ginger, Grated
5. ½ Cup Ice
6. ½ Cup Pineapple Juice, Frozen

Directions:

1. Just blend everything together and drink. Add ore ginger if your headache is really bad. You can even freeze your pineapple if you want a thicker consistency. If you're looking for a sweeter smoothie, then make sure to add raw honey.

www.ingramcontent.com/pod-product-compliance
Lightning Source LLC
Chambersburg PA
CBHW071245020426
42333CB00015B/1639